BEING FAT IS NOT OK
How to get the right mindset to finally lose weight and change your life

I0447982

Introduction

This book doesn't promise immediate results. It doesn't include miracle diets either. It doesn't include step-by-step plans for losing 40 pounds in a week.

So what the hell did I buy it for? You're probably asking yourself now.

Well, this book will help you understand why you are in the situation you are in, and change it. From my experience and that of many people I've met throughout all these years, I know that real change starts from inside, and the words you have in your hands right now will give you all the tools to begin that change.

The first step is to start reading it, of course, the second is to finish it, and then you're going to be on your way. It won't be easy but it will be very rewarding.

I have nothing more to say than to invite you to turn the page and start.

Ah! And of course, I would love you to join the Facebook community Being Fat is Not Ok, where you will find all the articles referred to in this book, and many others that will help you along this path.

The fattest woman in the world

Mayra Rosales sprang to fame in 2008 when she was arrested for allegedly killing her 2-year-old nephew. In her confession, she claimed that the child had died when, unintentionally, she had fallen on him, crushing his body. At the time, she was 28 years old and weighed 1000 pounds. She was considered the heaviest woman in the world.

The coroner's investigations determined almost immediately that Mayra had lied. The poor boy had actually been murdered by his mother, Jaime Lee Rosales, sister of the defendant, who had repeatedly beat him on the head with a brush, for refusing to eat. The original defendant was declared innocent and her sister was finally sentenced to 15 years in prison after being arrested in Mexico.

Why did Mayra Rosales lie? She argued at first that she had done it out of love for her sister, but when questioned further, the real reasons emerged. "I was alive, but I didn't live life. I thought I was dying anyway, so I decided to confess the murder to protect my sister."

Six years have passed since that incident, which appeared on every TV show and went around the world. Today, Mayra Rosales weighs 200 lbs. After her sister's conviction, she decided that she had to live a healthier life to be able to take care of her remaining nephews, who suddenly had no mother. She began an incredible process that allowed her to lose almost 800 lbs, which included 11 surgeries, but also a different way of thinking about food and her health in general.

"The way I see food now is that I have to eat to live. Before I was living to eat, and now, you know, I have a normal way of focusing on it. I'm not diabetic (anymore), I don't have high cholesterol, I don't have high blood pressure", she stated recently in an interview on ABC Nightline.

Trimming all that weight not only changed her life as far as health was concerned. Before the macabre incident of 2008 she had spent years sitting in a bed because she couldn't walk; today she has an Instagram account with more than 18,000 followers, in which she publishes photos of her body, gives health advice and even boasts about her new boyfriend. Not only she's alive, she has begun to live.

Of course, like the vast majority of those who begin to read this book, you must be thinking right now. "I don't weigh 1000 pounds! I'm just a little overweight." But, believe me, your story has much more in common with Mayra's than you think.

The double-edged sword of society

Turn on your television. In the first channel you tune, choose any show you like. No matter which one you've chosen, you will surely see attractive men and women. If you wait a bit for commercials to appear, it will probably be worse. Well-formed bodies, perfect faces, maximum confidence.

Does it cause you discomfort? To a lot of my friends, it does, especially to women. It irritates them immensely that society puts these people as role models. "Normal people are not like that!" They protest, especially in social networks. "The characters we see on television, in the movies and in the ads shouldn't look like that!"

They are partly right. The massification of the media has caused the world to surrender to the model of Western beauty, to an ideal of slim women and men, with perfect teeth and radiant hair. If you or me tried to be like that, we probably couldn't. And it's normal for people to be frustrated.

The problem is that, even while being normal, these people are taking the wrong approach. To understand this, we first have to understand the reality that surrounds the people who appear on television and in advertisements.

To begin with, I will give you an example. I'm sure many of you like sports. You probably have an idol, someone who plays at a level that very few can reach. Surely you have also practiced that same sport, maybe when you were a kid, hopefully you still do it now. Have you ever dreamed of being like your idol? I am convinced that you have. Did you succeed? I know not, because you probably wouldn't be reading this book. Did that generate an enormous amount of frustration to you? I really doubt it. I don't know anyone who said, "Why tennis matches on TV are not played by normal people instead of Roger Federer or Serena Williams!"

And that is the lesson to be learned. The women and men who appear in advertisements and movies are professionals. Their job is to be beautiful, and in the case of models and actors their future depends on staying slim and being able to look sexy in front of the camera. To achieve this, on many occasions they must perform extraordinary sacrifices, rigorous diets, strenuous training and, in many cases, plastic surgeries. And not only that, they usually have other people around them that help sell that fantasy of perfection. Photographers who choose the ideal light and precise angle; expert makeup artists to correct the imperfections of a face and highlight its most attractive features; graphic designers who apply a good dose of Photoshop to their pictures and videos to remove the imperfections that these models share with any ordinary person. Many times, when you see them in person, you wonder if they are really the same ones that appear in the ads. The world of fashion is in equal measure illusion and reality.

Therefore, don't think that those who appear in commercials and television shows are called 'models' because they are role models. They are simply people like any other who have a job, with the difference that their job is to look as attractive as possible. A profession that neither you nor I have, so it's absurd to become obsessed with imitating them. It's not worth it.

To give you an idea, let me use an example. Just a few days ago I read an Esquire magazine article called "The Rise and Rise of the spornosexual". On it, reporter Max Olesker describes the process that he had to follow to have a Spornosexual body, which, in his own words, is:

"A more extreme breed of man than his metro(sexual) forebear. He is just as plucked, tanned and moisturised, but leaner, buffer, more jacked and obsessed not just with "looking good" in the abstract, but with the actual physical proportions of his frame: the striation of his abs, the vascularity of his biceps, the definition of his calves.
He defines himself less by the clothes he wears than by his HD-ready body, which is perpetually ready to be ogled on the beach, admired on the high street as it bursts out of a skin-tight plunging V-neck T-shirt, or rubbed-up-against under the flickering strobe of an Essex nightclub. He was defined as the

"modern British douchebag" by writer Clive Martin in Vice, who described him as "an erection in a vest. A walking, preening monument to the British masculinity crisis, a sports science Übermensch with an indecent exposure charge to his name."

Let's say it's the type of body that Hugh Jackman and Cristiano Ronaldo have, although the most usual examples given are Brad Pitt in The Fight Club and Edward Norton in American History X. Incredibly muscular, but not huge, and without an ounce of fat.

To get this body, Olesker, a guy with a totally normal complexion, had to dedicate himself full-time three months to a program that included a personal trainer and an extremely rigorous diet. After a while, the reporter described his daily life.

"Two-thirds of the way through my training regime, I am constantly exhausted, constantly sore, and constantly going either to or from the gym. My whole life becomes governed by

an immutable set of weekly edicts issued by (his personal trainer) Walker. I buy Tupperware containers and begin to weigh each of my five daily high-protein meals, then log them for his approval on the My Fitness Pal app, as per his orders. Walker tells me I "no longer eat breakfast. From now on, think of it as 'Meal One'." On some days, my 'Meal One' consists of chicken and spinach. Alcohol is verboten in this new world, as are carbohydrates. As is sugar. As is fruit. I am restricted to one coffee per day. My strict adherence to the times I must eat means that I find myself hastily consuming meals while on the bus, outside in the street and, on one particularly low occasion, standing on the eastbound Central Line platform at Oxford Circus tube station (subway stations in England)".

At the end of the period, Olesker achieved his goal, and the before and after photos of the article are impressive. But what was his feeling on the last day?

"The "after" photos are taken. I feel relief, more than anything else. I have achieved what I set out to — I have transformed myself as best I could — but I realized the thing that makes me happiest of all is that very soon I'll be allowed to eat some bread. It's a good feeling".

If they asked me, "would you like to look like this?" The answer would be "of course!" But if the next question were, "would you be willing to sacrifice your entire life for it?" The answer would be, "no way!" I have other priorities, and I understand that it would simply be an unattainable ideal for my situation, so I don't obsess about what society considers a perfect body.

The other side of the coin

"I am beautiful, no matter what they say. Words can't bring me down." In 2002, Christina Aguilera made this song the hymn of self-acceptance. The song was actually composed by Linda Perry who, a few years before, was also a famous singer with the group Four Non Blondes. They are both right, we are all beautiful.

That doesn't mean, however, that we all feel beautiful, and it's a very important difference. In recent years, we have experienced a strange dichotomy. On one hand, society constantly parades handsome men and women on the screens in front of us but, on the other hand, we live in a world that has become politically correct to the extreme, and that part of society tells us "if you are overweight, it doesn't matter, you are beautiful too." And that, unfortunately, is not true.

At this moment, I want to make a pause, to make clear one of the most important concepts in this book. In my opinion, beauty and health are closely related. I believe that, beyond the outside looks, what make a person beautiful are her habits and her way of life. The reason is simple, a healthy person is usually a person who feels good about herself, who conveys a positive energy that transcends her physical traits, and who positively effects those around her.

An insecure person, who struggles to accept her appearance and who knows she could look and feel better, radiates a very different energy. And unfortunately, on many occasions, that happens at both ends of the body mass spectrum.

We had already talked about one of the contradictions in today's society, now let's talk about another. Usually, when we see an extremely thin person, we immediately assume that she is ill, and we conclude that she might have an eating disorder. Countless images of other people in the same situation pass through our minds. When we see an overweight person, however, the feeling is very different. Unless the amount of extra pounds is huge, it seems normal to us. We all have friends or acquaintances like that, or maybe it's us who have an obesity problem and to see another overweight person no longer surprises us, but it shouldn't be that way.

This is not intended to be a technical book, but I'll give you a few statistics so that you realize why being overweight, despite being a major problem, has been normalized by society.

Until the twentieth century, one of the biggest problems of the human race in general was malnutrition, to the point that having a few extra kilos was seen as a symbol of status. Paul Rubens, one of the great artists of the Renaissance, painted several large-format paintings of Marie de Medici, the Queen of France, showing her in this way.

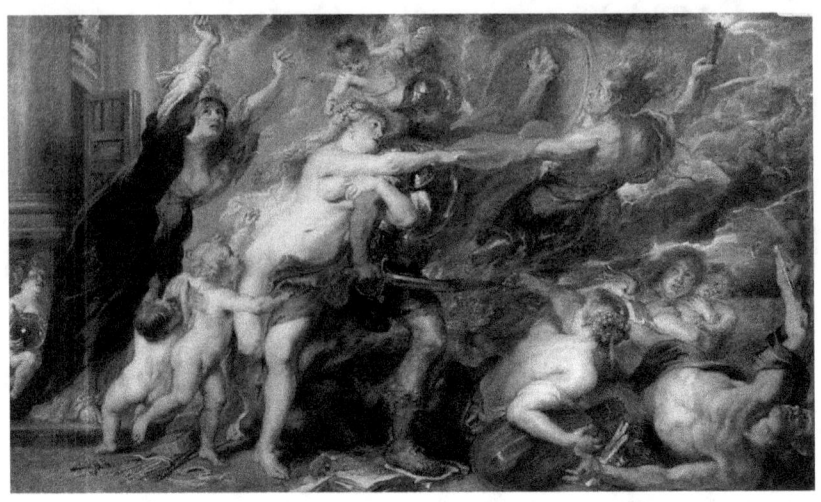

And this is his painting of the Greek god Bacchus, who even

being the patron of food and drink, would certainly not be

represented by an artist in this way nowadays.

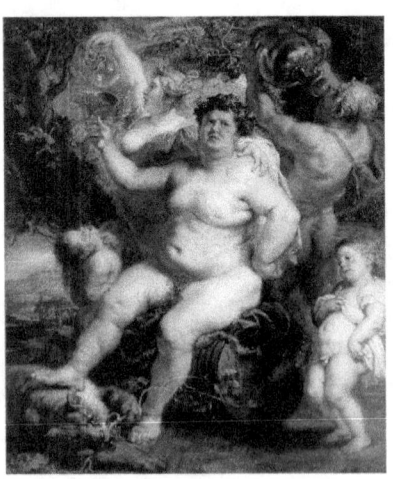

However, from the second half of the twentieth century on the situation began to change, especially in developed countries. The technological revolution made it possible to increase the quantity of food available to regular people and lowered its price, to the point that, in just a century, eating habits had completely changed. As an example, in 1909 the average American ate 4 pounds of cheese a year, by 2000 cheese consumption had increased eightfold to 32 pounds a year![1]

The situation became more dramatic with the passage of time, in 1962, 13% of people in the United States were obese and 45% were overweight. By 2012, 30% are obese and 74.1% are overweight. And, according to figures from the World Health Organization, 500 million people suffer from obesity around the planet.

We are done. No more statistics. Promised. (Okay, there will be one more, a little later but it will be the last one). I just wanted to give you an idea of the magnitude of the problem and why it seems increasingly common to see overweight people around us. After all, 7 out of 10 is far from a small number!

Thus, society has normalized "gaining a few extra pounds", to the point that, when we see others, we don't really realize they're overweight at all! The problem is that we're deceiving ourselves, and not just that; we know that we are deceiving ourselves. How can I say this with complete certainty? It's easy. When we see an overweight person we are not surprised, but when we see ourselves in the mirror and notice that we look fatter than before, or if we try to wear clothes that we bought a year ago and no longer fit us, then we panic or get depressed. When we talk about weight, we are willing to let go of what happens around us, but when it comes to ourselves, it affects us immediately.

If one does a search on Amazon using the word "diet", the amount of books is impressive. Today, December 16, 2016, the number is 28,639. And many of them have titles that describe the feelings of those who overeat. "Letting go of Bad Habits, Guilt and Anxiety", "Change your Lifestyle Without

Suffering", "Reclaim your Energy and Focus, Upgrade your Life". It's clear that, at least as far as weight is concerned, "I am beautiful, no matter what they say" is a lie. Maybe we are, but this is not how we feel, and the solution is not trying to convince ourselves that being overweight is okay, but to do something about it. And that's what this book is all about.

My little story of ups and downs

I'm going to make a confession. I am not overweight. In fact, I've hardly ever being in my life. When I was a child, it was rather the opposite, I was extremely thin. Despite eating sweets and drinking soft drinks without any restraint, my weight never increased even a pound. As a teenager, one night I woke up thirsty and I drank five cans of apple soda, one after another, I didn't complete the six-pack because, in the middle of the sixth, I felt guilty and left it for the next day.

In my twenties, the pattern remained the same. I didn't eat so badly, but I didn't take much care of myself. Of course, I never smoked and drank very little so all the calories I ate came from food, and although my diet was never very healthy, it was not bad enough to actually gain weight. Besides, I always practiced sports. Football and tennis, at least once a week, sometimes more, and also used to run from time to time.

For years and years, my weight remained about 175 pounds, sometimes a little more, sometimes a little less, a totally normal number for my height of 6 feet. My body was the least of my worries, although I must admit that I sometimes saw TV actors and thought, "it would be nice to have a body like that!" But I did nothing to actually get it.

Then something strange happened. One day that I didn't have anything to do, I switched on the television. There was a show called "Extreme Makeover," a reality show in which men and women underwent a series of fixes to improve their appearance. Most of them were surgeries but, in the end, they spent a few months dieting and working out with a personal trainer whose name, if I remember correctly, was Michael Thurmond.

The part of the hundred surgeries seemed repulsive and artificial, but the the training and diet one captivated to me from the beginning. What would happen if I submitted myself to something like that? I was very curious and I wanted to try. The problem is, back then I didn't have enough discipline. I remember buying Thurmond's diet book and convincing my then girlfriend that we should try to follow it together. One day before we started, she chickened out and decided not to start. That broke my determination and in the end I didn't do it either. In the book there were also some workout routines but they were almost all with elastic bands and I got bored by the second day. In the end, I bought some weighs and every morning I did a little workout in my house, but without a clear idea of what I wanted to do or which need I wanted address. After a few months, I abandoned that too. My first attempt had completely failed, but the seeds were planted for what would happen next.

A few years later, I changed city and country. I wanted to start a new life and that included going to a gym for the first time, so I signed up for a very small one that was near my new home. Very happy, I arrived the first day and began to use the machines. As I did, I saw that a very muscular man would not stop looking at me. After half an hour, he came to me and said, "Hi, I'm one of the monitors of the gym, sorry to intrude, but you're not doing your exercises the right way, and I want to keep you from having an injury."

I felt pride clouding my eyes, who was this guy to tell me what to do? But the sensation only lasted a second and then common sense prevailed. Not only he was the gym monitor, but also someone with a much better trained body than mine. He had to know something that I didn't so, swallowing every ounce of my vanity, I asked him what I should do.

He wrote a specific routine for what I wanted at that time (gain muscle) and he explained the correct technique for each of the exercises. Before he left, he told me something that would change my life. "I saw the weight you were trying to lift, it was definitely too little for your body type. You have to learn to stretch your limits. To get what you want, you should always try to go further. Here in the gym, always try to increase the weight you lift, at least a little every day. You have to leave here feeling that your today self is at least a little better than your yesterday self."

I must admit that my discipline in that gym lasted only a few months. My job at the time required a lot of time and the change of cities caused me to meet many new people and start a more active social life, so I stopped going. But more seeds were sown and one day they would germinate.

Over the next few years, as I grew older, I began to worry more about my appearance. I bought better quality clothing and researched basic fashion concepts. I must admit that I even exaggerated at times, and spent a lot of money on something that now seems excessive, but now, analyzing it, I think it had to do with a real concern about aging and the desire to maintain a good image. I unconsciously sought to feel better about myself and, without much idea of how, and, in a rather disorganized way, I tried to do something about it.

Then, by chance, I discovered Tim Ferriss's book, "The 4-Hour Body". I will not say that it changed my life, because the signs were already there long before, but it did help me to picture a clearer path. The slow-carbohydrate diet it proposed was ideal for the things I liked to eat and represented a challenge. Besides, it looked a lot like what I had seen in Extreme Makeover so many years back. I liked less the exercise routines of the book so I decided not to apply that part, but, more for self-experimentation than anything else, I decided to start his diet, very shortly after I finished the book.

As I told you, since I left my teenage years, my weight was always around 175 pounds, and the truth is that I didn't feel uncomfortable with my body, but obviously there was something in my head that pushed me to do it. The experiment lasted 8 months, in which I lost 15 pounds. If I was thin before, when I decided to stop the diet I didn't have an ounce of fat! I did it without starving myself at all too, because the slow-carb diet allows you to eat all the meat and vegetables you want. Of course, I must admit that at first it was difficult for me to leave sweets, but after a while I got used to it.

It's funny because now, when I see pictures of those days, I realize that I was exaggeratedly thin, but in those times it made me happy to wear an S-sized shirt, or pants a size smaller than usual. I think it had to do with what the gym instructor had said back then, that every day I had to push myself a little more, and I applied that advice to the diet.

8 months passed and new changes arrived to my life. After many years as a freelancer, I got a stable job, with a fixed schedule, and that caused my days to become more predictable. In addition, I moved house again. It was then that I thought it was time to do something I had postponed for many years: to go back to the gym, but this time for real.

I signed up for one that was near my new flat, where it was necessary to have a session with an instructor to start a routine according to your needs. That day I explained to him that I wanted to gain muscle and he wrote the exercises that he thought would be best for that.

During the following year, I went to the gym five days a week, always trying to do the exercises with the proper technique and gradually increasing the weight. I also completely changed my diet. I started to eat double or triple what I ate before I started going to the gym and gradually incorporated carbohydrates into my diet. I also researched on the Internet what supplements could be useful without being harmful to my health, and I started to take them, although in the end I only stayed with meat protein powder.

The result was that I added 11 pounds of muscle to my frame and completely changed its shape. My genetics didn't allow me to have a six-pack but other than that, I got the body I had always wanted.

In any diet book or makeover TV show this would be a happy ending, but that's not how life works. There came a time when I got sick of so much discipline and started going to the gym less and less. In addition, I left my stable job; I began to have a more active social life, to drink more and to eat desserts every day. And although my body held strong for quite some time, the consequences finally arrived.

My usual job is journalism, and that includes recording videos for social networks. About six months ago, because I was traveling, I had to record one of those videos sitting down instead of standing up and the result left me in shock, I had gained a lot of weight! It also didn't help when I told my mother and my girlfriend and neither of them replied, "it's not true, you look great". The truth was there for everyone to see.

That was a new wake-up call, I went back to the diet, right away, and as soon as I could, I re-entered the gym. Three months later, I was back in my normal weight, 178 pounds, and I then decided that the time to be radical was over.

Now I play tennis twice a week, I go to the gym two more days, and eat what I like, but without excesses. I have learned that the most important thing is to feel good, even if I don't have a perfect body, but that I must also pay attention not to exceed myself. And it's the message I want to convey to you.

Before closing this chapter I want to share with you what I learned during all these years, and that forms the basis of this book.

- It doesn't matter if you are overweight or not, we are all exposed to feeling self-conscious about our bodies, and that can always reach extremes.

- Often, real changes come in the form of wake-up calls or, as I call them, "enough is enough moments", where you say "stop", and modify your habits immediately.

- No matter which regime or diet you follow, the important thing is to find a program that suits your needs and tastes.

- Always try to be better than the previous day, in everything.

- Change is never easy and it always takes time, but with discipline and dedication, results can be achieved.

- The most difficult thing is always to start. In my opinion, the period of adaptation for a new change is 3 weeks, afterwards the body ceases to resist and adapt to their new reality.

- It is possible to fall, and there is no happy ending. We must try to have several "happy endings". There will be stages in life when our weight will fluctuate, but it is important to set a limit and know that this limit should not be exceeded.

- To be radical is to good to begin with, but once the first goal is achieved, we must know how to find a balance. We don't necessarily need to leave the things we like to do if we find suitable alternatives. For example, I like to eat chocolate, and don't want to sacrifice that now, so I prefer to workout more and not to deprive me of one of my pleasures.

- When working out, you have to find activities that allow you to have fun. In my case going the gym and playing tennis. Doing things because "it's my duty", is always a losing proposition.

- The most important thing, always, is to feel good, physically and mentally. It's not necessary to aspire to the perfect body or to imitate anybody. We should be our only reference.

Kereem's story

I already told you my story. And maybe you're thinking, "But if he has never been overweight, how would he know my problems?" I would like to think that, after my tale, you might have realized that we all have the same problems, and that, in my case, although they didn't show in the same way, I had the same insecurity feelings as you do.

But don't worry. To show you that I know what I'm talking about, and that the change of mentality that I'm describing applies to everyone, I want to introduce you to Kereem.

Kereem is one of my best friends, and since he suffered a traumatic situation at age 20, he has been overweight. Now he's 29 and he's finally getting his body and mind in order. It took him 9 long years and a lot of learning and I'm sure that in the story that he will share, you will find many points in common with what has happened in your life.

"Before I was 20, I was an athletic young man. I had never had problems with being overweight even though my diet was really bad: I ate everything in large quantities and also drank a lot of cola. To counter, I spent most of my days in soccer training sessions and playing with friends from my block. That's why, despite not taking any care of myself, my weight was around 145 pounds. Not bad for a 5.8 feet boy.

When I started college, my eating habits worsened. Between classes and social life I had little time to cook healthy food. This resulted in me spending my days eating pizza, hot dogs, hamburgers and all kinds of fast food. And of course, there was not enough time to do the same amount of exercise as when I was in high school.

Little by little I was gaining weight, but I didn't worry too much. True, I had to buy clothes a couple of sizes larger, but the situation was not serious enough to notice. There was my first failed attempt at something like a diet. Without any real knowledge behind it, my instinct -and my friends- recommended changing fast food for salads.

I also tried to take advantage of the fact that there was a free gym at the university to start an exercise routine and take my body from flaccid to muscular, like that of the athletes who trained there.

I failed.

The pain of the first few days, as well as the extra effort for exercise, made me start eating more. Gradually I stopped going to the gym, but I kept the amount of food I was eating. I was also partying and drinking a lot. In consequence, little by little, my weight kept going up.

Fortunately, even if it wasn't intense, my level of physical activity was enough to maintain a relatively acceptable weight. During my first two years of college I always managed to stay close to 175 pounds. I was overweight, but not so much.

The real problem came after the second year. Due to economic problems, I had to leave school. Well, they actually kicked me out. At the same time, the girl I was dating left me for another guy and not just that, she kept the flat we were renting together. For a couple of days I had to sleep on the street, before moving back with my parents. This, I find it hard to admit, made me really sad. So I sought immediate refuge from my pain and found it in food.

I spent almost a year in a deep depression. Twelve months that could be summarized this way: waking up, eating, playing video games, eating more, lying on my bed, eating again and going back to sleep. I ate whatever I had nearby whether it was healthy or not. And I always accompanied my meals with a big bottle of cola.

So I passed from being slightly overweight to obese. I started to go to a psychologist but, by the time the therapy had taken effect and I was again in a much better state of mind, my weight was close to 245 pounds.

Looking at myself in the mirror was a horrible experience. I didn't recognize the person who was in front of me. But it was even worse to enter a store and not to be able to buy anything because even the larger sizes were too tight for me. Or even worse, that I could find something that fit but looked terrible because of the shape of my body. That dampened my mood again and I took refuge in food one more time. It was a vicious circle.

Until that point I hadn't tried any diet to lose weight. I thought that I would have the same body for the rest of my life and while I tried to accept it, I actually hated it. Feel-better slogans and advertising campaigns made me feel even worse. "Be happy as you are", they said, or "embrace your body", how could I be happy or embrace something I didn't like? I challenge those people who came up with these things to stand before the mirror and look like a ball of fat as I did. Then they could give me advice!

I didn't even have any idea who "those people" were. I was looking for a way out of my anger. I was wrong. Instead of blaming others I had to put myself to work.

Thanks to my great friend, Martin Langer, I started to take action to lose weight. I owe him much of what I am today because he not only convinced me to start dieting but also encouraged me to finally take action.

The diet he showed me is called "The Slow-Carb Diet". Tim Ferriss explained it in his book "The 4-Hour Body". It's pretty simple: you can't eat sugar, starches, pasta, fruit or anything that has simple carbohydrates.

Outside the forbidden foods, I could eat anything, as much as I wanted. It was the perfect diet for me, as I love to eat. And it worked. For the first time I lost weight.

From 245 pounds I managed to be just above 210. I was finally happy! I was still obviously overweight, but it was a great success. Unfortunately this brought to light another of my key problems: the lack of discipline.

After losing weight I started to loosen up on the diet. The result, of course, was a yo-yo effect. I was saddened, but it wasn't as hard as before. This time I knew that I had a tool to lose those pounds if I wished so.

And so a couple of extremely erratic years passed. I was down 30 pounds, then back up. I bought smaller clothes and a few weeks later had to buy bigger clothes. It was a mess, because without discipline I couldn't get anywhere.

I tried. I really tried. I added exercise to the diet. I worked out with the Insanity program several times. But history repeated itself: up and down, up and down. In the past it was school, now it was my job, I always had some excuse not to stick to a regime.

Europe changed everything. Fortunately for me, besides my weight issues, everything in my life was going much better and I could fulfill one of my dreams, getting a job in Barcelona. And it was there where my reality hit harder than I could have imagined.

I'm Mexican, and in my home city I never had a major problem to have some success with the girls I liked, despite being so *obviously overweight (Mexico is one of the countries with more obese people in the world). In Europe, the story was different. VERY different.*

Going out to the clubs in Barcelona and being ignored by 99 percent of girls there was one of the toughest experiences of my life. To talk to them and to be rejected after 2 minutes because of the way I looked still makes me cringe.

It's true, in a relationship what matters are the feelings that two people share. And girls love a good sense humor and an interesting personality. Of course, I understand all that, but in a club that always come second.

For starters, there were always more men than women, therefore a greater number of options for them. And between a good-looking guy that could make them laugh and a nice chubby guy with the same ability, the choice was quite simple.

This was difficult to assimilate. But the blow was strong enough to shake the foundations of my bad habits. I would change, even if it cost me tears of blood.

Again I turned to the excellent slow-carb diet, although I was not so strict at first. For my workout, I chose to run. I found it to be quite simple and I could gradually increase the pace. Everything was going great. I dropped from 210 pounds on average to 185-190, but then something unexpected happened.

I was working out without any knowledge or guidance and this, added to the excitement of starting to have success, made me abuse the capabilities of my body. I severely injured the soleus muscle of my right leg and I had to stop my activity for a couple of weeks.

That couple of weeks turned into months. I forgot to diet again and, until I saw myself in the mirror one afternoon, visiting a friend's house in Madrid, I didn't realize how deep I had fallen again.

I remember it as if it were yesterday. Standing in front of the mirror, staring at my round-shaped body and saying:

"You have just turned 29. You are less than 365 days away from the decade that, since childhood, you dreamt would be the best of your life. Right now, you're no different from that fat kid that was constantly depressed and never left the couch. You've changed many things on the inside and have a relatively good professional career, but deep down you are still that undisciplined and fragile child. You don't need tears of blood, you simply need to grow up and take responsibility for yourself. There should be no more excuses. From today you have a day less in the goal of starting your thirties in the best possible way."

And there, finally, a decade later, I began to behave the way I had imagined from the first time I set a foot on a gym. I started the diet again, to the letter. It was not easy because I was living in the house of a friend who loves junk food. I didn't care. I had a clear vision in my mind.

Beans, chicken, frozen vegetables. The first thing I thought was that I had to be as practical as possible to prevent my own laziness to sabotage my plans. If I could prepare simple and fast meals, I would be safe. I moved back to Barcelona and there, in addition to the diet, I started running again. This time, instead of wanting to run marathons in a week, I decided to take a much more serene pace. I wasn't going to be quick, I was going to be effective.

The result was that I got my weight back down to 195 pounds. Total bliss! But still far from the goal... Now it was time to tighten my belt instead of loosening it.

I began to watch, every day, at least a couple of transformation videos on Youtube. People with the same problems and how they overcame them. It was a little silly, perhaps, but very effective, especially for those days when laziness tried to convince me not to exercise. Today, I continue with this kind of motivation.

I kept my weight at 195 pounds, but I seemed to have reached a point where I couldn't lose more. It was time to add another type of physical activity. Again, I searched the Internet for *answers. I thought about going to a gym, do the Insanity*

program again, or maybe crossfit.

In the end I chose calisthenics, more by chance than anything

else. On Twitter I found people who challenged themselves to

do 22 push-ups a day for 22 days. I decided to give it a

try. Upon completion of the 22 days I changed the routine to

three sets of 20 push-ups. Through my research I understood

that to do it daily was not the best idea and I decided to make

it day in and day out.

There was no doubt, I had finally changed, but I needed much

better organization so that I could finally get the results I

wanted. With the help (again) of YouTube and various

publications, and taking advantage of having a park nearby

with the necessary equipment to practice, I stepped up in the

calisthenics, doing exercises with my own body weight.

I stopped running daily. Not out of laziness but by strategy. I

programmed my own beginner's routine and I went on my way

to get my best physical version before reaching 30.

So far it hasn't been an easy road, but it's true that I was my own worst enemy by filling it with obstacles myself. After nearly nine years of ups and downs, I have been working nonstop for the last six months. By now it has ceased to be an extra effort and has become my daily routine.

The diet has become an integral part of my life. It went from being an obligation and turned into my actual eating habits. In the past, passing in front a fast food joint provoked all sorts of cravings; today it doesn't excite me in the least. I still enjoy eating, of course, but in a much more rational way.

Almost 180 days after that tough talk with myself, I can say with joy that my weight is down to 165-170 pounds. I'm a thin man. I notice, my friends notice. The girls in clubs notice it. I feel good. I like what I see in the mirror, not just the reflection, but also because I know all the work behind it.

My attitude has changed. I am a much more confident person. It partly has to do with my body; I won't lie, but also and by large with discovering the ability to dominate myself and get rid of my urges. It gives you power, lets you see that you can achieve anything you set your mind to, as long as you're willing to work for it with intelligence and discipline.

Today, I understand much more those campaigns that ask you to accept yourself as you are. They're right, but not in the way most people see them. In my talk with myself, the day I really changed my life, the first step I had to take was to accept me as I was. To see my shortcomings and what they had done to my body. The exterior was a reflection of the interior.

Before saying goodbye I want to share with you what I learned over the years.

- *You must begin by accepting yourself. By really seeing things the way they are and knowing that it's in your hands to change them. You have the power to transform yourself.*
- *Enthusiasm is temporary, discipline lasts forever. You have to be strict with yourself, go out to exercise even on days when you don't feel upbeat and keep your diet*

even if you crave to break it and go get that burger around the corner (although you can always have a cheat day to be able to satisfy those cravings).

- *Less is more. Start exercising slowly and increase it as time passes. That's a much more effective strategy than doing extreme routines or challenges far beyond your ability.*

- *Everything changes one step at a time. You may not notice changes right away, but they're happening all the time. Every step you take in the direction of the goal you set to yourself brings you closer to it.*

- *Measuring and weighing is critical. Check your weight every day and the seventh day take an average of the week. That same day take measurements of your body and keep a record. That way the changes will be more evident to you.*

- *Find an exercise or sport you enjoy. It can be swimming, running, skiing, etcetera. In my case it was running and doing calisthenics. The important thing is that you enjoy it so you don't leave it.*

- *Use everything you can to motivate yourself daily. Watch videos on YouTube, paste pictures on your room walls, listen to podcasts, whatever. Constantly feed on this type of stimulus to keep going. It's very important.*

Being Fat is Not Ok

I think Kereem's story is quite clear. It's time to stop fooling ourselves. Being overweight is not good. I am aware that there is a part of society that insists that there's no problem, that any form of body is acceptable, but I'm sure that deep inside your heart you know that being fat is not ok and you want to do something about it.

I would not, however, want you to think this is just my opinion, so in this section I gathered some of the best insights I've found on the net about the subject, and I think they synthesize perfectly why it's time to set aside political correctness and tell ourselves that the world is not doing us a favor by telling us that being overweight is natural, much less beautiful.

The first text I will mention appeared on the website SparkNotes and was written in 2014 by the English user rawrdinosaurr. It's called "Why we need to stop pretending being overweight is fabulous", and I'll quote something that I found very interesting, because it explains why the message of "we are all beautiful" can't be true from an evolutionary point of view.

"You may cry 'But love doesn't judge! Everybody is beautiful!' However, the very idea of beauty centers on the fact that not everyone can be beautiful. It's as simple as that - if everyone were beautiful, then no one would be. It takes all meaning out of the word…

I suppose I should define what it really means to be attractive. To be attractive is to possess qualities that are desirable in a reproductive partner. The same principle applies to animals - survival of the fittest, with the fittest being the most attractive. This doesn't necessarily mean the quickest runners; it just means those best adapted to survive…

In the modern world, money helps you to survive; hence it is an attractive quality. In (the past), wealth often manifested itself as obesity, as rich people could afford to buy more food, and enjoy it more, eating a rich diet…

Nowadays, though, most people in the developed world can afford to feed themselves, and the focus is no longer on this in terms of the manifestation of wealth.

Overweight people are more likely to die young - hence they are less likely to survive, and are not the best adapted. So obesity has fallen out of favor, things such as high-powered jobs have replaced it.

You may say, 'so what? I can be as fat as I like, and I don't care if people don't like it. Besides, I'm overweight and I get plenty of dates. I love my curves.'… That's not what it's about. It feels nice to be thin - anyone who has lost lots of weight will tell you that - and a healthy weight for most people looks skinny. Not skin and bones (as being anorexically thin gives the impression - biologically speaking - that you can't feed yourself, so people might not find that attractive either), but not fatty either. Going back to our Darwinism, being thin and toned can also mean you are fit and athletic, strong and enduring - definitely beneficial characteristics. And do you really want the agonizing joint pain, shortness of breath and constant risk of *strokes, diabetes or heart attacks to worry about? Like it as*

not, obesity will shorten your life."

The article was interesting because it delves on two issues

that are fundamental aspects of this book. The first, and most

important, it is that being overweight is dangerous to your

health and therefore should be avoided. And the second is

that while it is true that we are all beautiful by the mere fact of

being alive and being good people, that doesn't mean that we

feel beautiful or that society sees us that way, and so I think it

was worth to quote the part that talks about why,

evolutionarily, obesity is no longer an attractive trait.

Of course, one thing is to say something like this and a

completely different one is to "body shame" someone. And I

think that's a practice that society should eliminate

altogether. To discriminate for any reason is wrong, whether

it's race, religion, sexual orientation and, of course, physical

appearance. But unlike all the others, being overweight is not

a natural characteristic of human beings and, in most cases, it's something that can be avoided with discipline and effort. I will never agree with those who criticize those who are different, but I can't stay silent about the irrational defense of something that is clearly harmful to health and that is essentially caused by ourselves (other than the ones with valid medical or psychological reasons, of course).

Therefore, the following text I will quote goes against the Fat Acceptance Movement. This movement, which emerged just a few years ago, suggests that, no matter how overweight we may be, we must consider it normal and equates its "struggle" with the ones that women, minorities and homosexuals have had to endure. In my opinion, this is absurd, an idea shared by the site tips.straighthealth.com, on a post on their blog published in June 5, 2012, from which I will quote some excerpts.

"These groups have a lot in common. They all equate their struggle with the civil rights movement. They mistakenly and offensively compare discrimination against Blacks with their

own "struggle" to live an unhealthy lifestyle. There's a huge difference between being denied basic human rights because of race or religion and fat people's struggle with being accepted by society for their unhealthy lifestyle choices. If they can't see the difference between being denied the right to vote because of skin color and being ridiculed because of size (which is completely under their control), then there might not be any hope for them after all. In addition to claiming fat acceptance as a civil rights issue, these groups also attempt to justify their obesity in a few ways. They call it beautiful, a personal choice and even healthy.

The most important similarity between the fat acceptance groups is their goal. Their goal isn't to help obese people fix themselves, it's the exact opposite. Instead of improving health and living conditions, they're working to show that obesity isn't a problem and therefore needs no fixing. Everyone agrees that it would be much easier to live a life void of any exercise or healthy food. Most of us would love to eat junk all day, never go to the gym and totally ignore our health, but living in lala land and pretending that all of that is somehow OK is a disservice to ourselves, friends & family and even society. That's why most of us know that being fat is bad. It's the same reason that smoking, drinking excessively and using recreational drugs is also frowned upon.

The main goal of these groups is to make fat people oblivious to the choices they're making. It's a lot easier to stay fat than it is to accept you're wrong and change. By pretending that fat can be healthy, they're enabling obese people to be lazy, eat junk food and live unhealthy lives. The civil rights movement was about empowering people, not blinding them.

Rather than trying to get society to accept obesity and sickness, these groups should be working to decrease obesity levels. Decreasing obesity levels would help improve the quality of life for millions of people, extend life expectancy and decrease health costs. Instead, these groups are doing just the opposite. They're giving obese people an excuse not to change by convincing them that fat is healthy, beautiful and normal. Being obese isn't normal, it's a condition that causes disease and lowers life expectancy.

The reason that this movement is becoming popular is because change isn't easy. Losing weight and starting a healthy lifestyle is hard, but staying unhealthy is even harder. In the short term, it's much easier to live a sedentary lifestyle and eat unhealthy junk food. Over time, this "easy" lifestyle will turn into frequent doctor trips, a regular diet of prescription drugs and extended hospital stays. You can avoid all of that if you start changing now. Realize that changing your own lifestyle is a lot easier and more rewarding than trying to force society to change its view."

I think the text explains quite well why it's healthier to try to change than "to accept yourself as you are", regardless of whether "being you" means being extremely overweight. I think it's very important to try to be happy with yourself, to look at the mirror and think "today I look good!" and not to receive constant blows to your self-esteem. And by that I don't mean anyone body-shaming you but rather the blows inflicted by yourself, because, ultimately, the only person we cannot fool is ourselves and when we can't button those pants, or when we have trouble climbing stairs, or when we realize that there are no sizes available for us in clothing stores, we know that something is not right, despite insisting otherwise.

Ultimately, no one, absolutely no one who has stopped being overweight has regretted it. In general, the stories we know, from friends and family or the ones that we have read on the Internet, always talk about how ecstatic the person was when she could finally shed those extra pounds that were burdening her for ages.

That brings us to the ultimate source of this chapter, the one that inspired this book's name. The famous viral video called "Being fat is not ok ... deal with it". In it, its author, YouTuber Richard Masucci, a clearly overweight 34-year old man, talks about how it's time to stop with the excuses and lies, and to make an effort to lose weight.

For a long time I hesitated whether to include it in the book or not. The reason is that, although it's a truly inspiring video, eight months after its publication, Masucci hasn't seem to have lost even a pound. His idea was to show a new "Richard" in May 2017 and, for the moment, December 2016 Richard seems to be much closer to the one that originally recorded the video.

In the end, I decided to include it because it still has very important things to say, and I think his ideas are worth taking into account, although he hasn't exactly followed them.

The video is more than 6 minutes long, so I will just transcribe here what seems to me are its most important phrases.

"I'm going to let you in on a secret. Being fat is not fucking okay! It's not healthy. It's not a race, it's not a religion, it's not a sexual preference – you are not well.
It shouldn't be accepted because it's a physical health condition that you have…
Now of course I'm not talking about people have different body types and there are some people who have a predisposition to be slender no matter what they eat. There are people that are going to have a couple of pounds in them no matter how

healthy they eat. I'm not talking about them – I'm not saying

everybody has to have washboard abs...

To the people who say that they have tough upbringings,

psychological disorders, whatever the case might be. I can

empathize with that, but at the same time people who are

slender have those issues too... you can't use that as a crutch

to say 'you know what, because of what I've been through,

this is why I'm fat and this is why I'm going to stay this way'.

Because your body doesn't give a shit! It doesn't say 'because

you were abused when you're a kid, I'm not gonna let you

have a clogged artery, because you were abused when you're

a kid, I'll pass on giving you the diabetes'. It's not healthy!

Wouldn't you want to live longer so you can enjoy a better part

of your life, when you got past the other bullshit that maybe

your mother or you father put you through?

I just don't understand, and I'll be the first to say, I have no

excuses for being the size I am except that I enjoy food. I'm

not unhappy, I'm not sad at all, I'm not depressed, I used to

have anxiety but honestly it has been next to none for the last

three years. To be honest to you, I just like to eat, and it's no excuse. Because, what's is going to have an extra bowl of cereal or an extra hamburger going to do for me besides make me feel like shit physically and get me to put me in an early grave".

As you can see, his words are really powerful. It's no coincidence that on the different platforms it was published, the video has had more than a million views, and has been reproduced by several major media around the world. After all, it's not the same to be lectured about weight by Men's Health magazine than by a 200-pound man.

Best of all were the comments to the video. As you may know, normally, on YouTube (and other social networks), every time you touch a controversial topic, comments from users may become offensive, aggressive and even cruel. In this case, however, most of them were rather supportive, and even several people said to have been inspired by Masucci's words to try to make a change in their lives and leave obesity behind.

And that is why, in the end, I decided to include the video on these pages. Because beyond the circumstance that the author has managed to overcome his own problems or not, if his experience inspired others to become better versions of themselves, then the video can be considered a success.

Truths and lies of the dieting world

In the two testimonies of this book, Kereem's and mine, we talked about Tim Ferriss "slow-carb diet", as the one best adapted to our needs. We both like to eat meat and we feel good with a protein-based diet.

That doesn't mean, however, that I recommend this diet as the only solution. This book is not about that and, as I have already mentioned and will do it again later, the whole philosophy of these pages is that there are many paths to reach the destination, as long as the basic principles are implemented.

In fact, I know many people for whom the slow-carb diet has not worked. In some cases because the type of food is not the one they like to eat and in others because, despite having followed it to the letter, they just wouldn't lose the weight they wanted.

In a few paragraphs I will explain in detail the eating habits I recommend, but let me talk to the world of diets.

One of the most important evidences that being overweight is not good is the amount of money that people spend to find solutions to their weight problems. According to a report from IBISWorld, the weight-loss industry raked in over 6 billion USD in 2015 with supplements selling several billion more. Weight-loss books occupy prominent places on the lists of best sellers on Amazon and there are entire shows dedicated to the subject on television.

The variety of diets, diet products, pills, books and options is endless, and as in any major industry, there are some that are very effective and others are outright fraud, and the vast majority are only effective if applied with discipline and rigor.

This book goes in that direction. The truth is that I don't care about which diet you use, as long as you commit to follow it. And you have understand a fundamental principle, therefore, that I'll put on a separate line and in larger letters:

There are no magic solutions.

To lose weight you need two things: effort and discipline. It's as easy as that. It won't be easy and won't be quick. The advantage is that you can start slowly, and the motivation you get when you start losing weight will always serve you as an incentive to move forward and try harder.

There are, however, some elementary principles which almost all diets share, and that I will list here. Even if it's the only thing you do, if you follow these 9 points, you will begin to lose weight.

1. Eat less

Reading it, you're probably thinking, "wow! What an amazing advice!" And yes, it is so obvious that it sounds indeed ridiculous. But think about it, how many times have you eaten more than you really need? How many times have you eaten only out of boredom? How many times have you eaten just because you have something nearby? No need to answer.

What I'm telling you here is that you should eat only what you need. When you feel satisfied, stop. And don't eat again until you're hungry. It sounds simple and I know that in practice it's not so much but the following points will help you to achieve it.

2. Eliminate sugar from your diet

It's as simple as that. Overall, this book has no strong recommendations. This book is about changing your mindset and it's not intended to give step by step instructions, but in this case I will be very clear: any attempt to lose weight has to be linked with an elimination or at least a substantial reduction in sugar.

What is the easiest way to do this? In principle, replace it with sweeteners. Yes, I know, surely you have read that sweeteners may be worse than sugar. The truth is that it's not true, at least not in the short term, and not for the purposes we are looking for. Believe me, in my experience and that of my acquaintances, the best way to relieve a sugar rush is with sugarless sweeteners.

Thus, replace soda with diet soda. Ideally drink water but I am aware that it is often too great a leap to start (although you should try Club Soda). Replace your sweet snacks for sugarless pills. Yes, I know they do not taste like your beloved chocolate, but your body will get used to them, I promise. One trick that has served me spectacularly is to mix peanut butter (no sugar added) with a tablespoon of caramel or chocolate from the Walden Farms brand, which produces zero-calorie substitutes for sweets and fatty foods. They don't taste the same, of course, but they are enough to trick your body, especially if you mix them with peanut butter.

My general recommendation is to go to a weightlifters' store and look for sugarless desserts. You'll be amazed at how many options you'll find.

3. Only have around the things that you actually want to eat

If you are overweight, you don't only eat when you're hungry. You do it also when you crave something, or to calm your anxiety, or because you saw an advertisement on TV, or just because you have it on hand.

In fact, many times, we eat what we eat because we have it close to us. If next door from the office there is a cafe that sells donuts, we buy one because it's within our reach, otherwise we wouldn't even think of it.

There are things we can't control, like the cafeteria outside the office, but there are others that we can, and one of them is the food we have at our disposal at home. Let's face it, if there is a chocolate bar on the shelf, we will eat it, if we have a beer or soda in the fridge, we will drink them, and if there is a slice of pizza on the table, we will devour it. It depends entirely on us not having those things within our reach.

Human beings are lazy by nature. If you don't have snacks around, you will think three times before going outside, walk ten minutes or take the car to get to the store and buy something sweet. You're just not going to do it. The key then is not to have them on hand.

When you go to the supermarket, do it with a precise list of what you want to buy and follow it to the letter, if you can ask for delivery groceries, much better. If you need snacks either way, make sure they are sugar-free and make sure you get ones that you actually like. As an example, every time I did my diet, I bought several boxes of cherry flavored Smints, a brand of sugarless pills that I loved. Maybe I spent a little more money than if I'd bought a chocolate bar but whenever I felt a sugar craving, I just popped a Smint into my mouth. It happened several times a day but I was always prepared. After a while, I got used to it, I almost never had those cravings anymore and, when they happened, I knew what to do.

4. Choose a diet program and follow it

Like I said several times, this book doesn't recommend any special diet. I think the best way to get results in anything you set your sight on is to enjoy the process as much as possible, not turn it into a torture. Consequently, I tell you that a certain diet is the one and only and that you have to follow it, regardless of your tastes, I'm condemning you to failure.

That doesn't mean I don't think you should choose a diet. In my experience, it's much easier to achieve your goals when you have a structure behind you. In this case, you have the enormous advantage of being able to choose the structure that you like, because, ultimately, with effort and discipline, anyone will pay off.

Only one caveat, choose one that makes sense. If a diet lets you eat chocolate three times a day and drink all the soda you want, then it most likely will be absolutely useless.

What diet to choose? To help you decide, I will quote the main points of an article on page the www.bodybuilding.com, called "How to choose the best diet for you", which I think has a good summary of the steps to choose the correct regime.

Ditch the popular definition of diet

Americans are obsessed with diets, but did you know that before the media butchered the word diet to more commonly mean "restricted eating for the purpose of weight loss," a diet was merely all and any foods consumed by a person? Before you form your own nutrition philosophy, it's important to first disassociate the word from a negative frame of mind.

Learn from all the different nutrition plans, even if you don't follow them

Trudging through this nutritional tar pit alone is enough to sink anyone into a tizzy, but when you look deeply into the nitty-gritty of each "one-true" diet plan, they're not as different as you think. Barring extreme ones (ahem, grapefruit diet), many popular diets—paleo, low carb, high fat, plant-based, and so on—share a few worthwhile common values that anyone looking for a sustainable nutrition plan can live by

Discover success with any way of eating

You've witnessed success among vastly different diets. Sometimes these diets deviate from the norm and still produce science-defying results. Vegans have been able to build muscle by staying vegan. People can mold insane physiques eating only twice per day... As you can see, a successful nutrition strategy can vary greatly... Listen to your body and question how you feel. I say TGIF, which stands for Tummy Grumbles, Ingest Food. Tune-in to your own hunger cues to have greater success in the long term.

Eat for your body type

Most people can be classified among three categories: ectomorphs, mesomorphs, and endomorphs. Depending on your body type, your diet setup will differ quite a bit from someone else. These are just general guidelines to help give you an idea of what your body expects:

- *Ectomorphs: High metabolism and higher tolerance to carbohydrates. In general, ectomorphs tend to do better on high carbohydrates, moderate protein and fat. Typically, ectomorphs resemble the build of lean and lanky long-distance runners.*

- *Mesomorphs: The most balanced of the three, mesomorphs can build muscle and maintain low fat levels. Their body likes a balance of carbs, fat, and protein.*

- *Endomorphs: Endomorphs are reminiscent of powerlifters who have a slower metabolism and tend to hang on to both muscle mass and fat. They do quite well on high fat and lower carbohydrate intake.*

Listen to your body

When you eat something that your body disagrees with, it bites back with unsavory symptoms—sometimes immediately.

In addition to relying on indicators like weight loss and body composition, be mindful of important markers such as energy level, mood, appetite, normal bodily functions (regular bowel movements and sleep, for example), and so on to see whether a particular diet is working for you.

If you feel miserable after eating lactose, you know to limit dairy products. If you don't feel right on a low-carb diet after a while, logic follows that you should rethink it.

Adjust things in small bytes

Once you gather personal data from your experiences, make small tweaks instead of drastic changes. Introducing or eliminating too many things at once will simply muddle what's working and what's not.

Reassess every so often

Every once in a while, a well-known saboteur called "life" rattles you out of your groove: You just had a baby, you just got married, your financial situation changed, or you've taken on more stress elsewhere. These are all instances that prompt *a re-evaluation of your current nutrition strategy. Will your strategy continue to work for you in this scenario with these new factors?*

5. If you can, talk to a nutritionist, but don't wait to start your diet

I'll say something that might disappoint you but, in my experience, most nutritionists are a fraud, and know as much as you or me. In recent years countless schools have emerged and they give degrees, but in fact the recipients don't have adequate preparation and don't really help.

As this book doesn't recommend any radical diet, my advice is to start today and calibrate your diet in time through trial and error. If something doesn't work, leave it and if it does, keep it.

Of course, if you have the time, money and a good recommendation, go see a nutritionist, but try to make sure he knows what he does. If he tries to force you to have food allergy tests, don't mind him. The best are those that measure you body fat index, ask your habits and your goals and design a personalized diet regime.

6. One day a week, relax

One of the main reasons why I always liked the slow-carb diet was because it allowed me to relax once a week and eat whatever I wanted. Tim Ferriss says there is a physical reason as well, according to him your metabolism speeds up and helps you lose even more weight, but in my experience the importance was really psychological. It helped me to feel that I was not a prisoner of the diet and gave me a date to look forward to. Just 5 days more to eat that delicious chocolate!

Talking to my friends and acquaintances, I discovered that the idea of having a day to relax is useful for other diets too, for the same reason. Unless you're really obese and your mission is to lose the most weight in the shortest possible time (in which case, yes, I recommend seeing a doctor before starting), to eat more freely for 24 hours won't really represent any drawback your diet, other than gaining a few ounces more for a couple of days.

Let's be clear, it can only be one day a week! The important thing here is to maintain a disciplined mindset. You can relax, yes, but within a predetermined scheme you know beforehand. It's not going to work if you say, "Well, I guess it's okay if I do this twice a week." The idea of this book, in general, is to give you the tools to keep yourself under control in a way that won't needlessly make you suffer, but it's up to you to be strong and achieve your goals.

7. You don't have to eat all the food on your plate

This seems silly, but it is not. If you order a dish in a restaurant, or if someone prepares something for you, you are by no means obligated to eat everything on the plate. When you feel satisfied, stop.

Similarly, you do not have to ask for larger portions in restaurants. I know you're probably used to, but I swear that although the difference in price between a medium and a large soda is not much, it is in calories. Same with French fries.

Eat only what is necessary to be satisfied and to feel good, you have no need to fill yourself up to the brim. It's not good for your weight and therefore to your health.

8. Research and adapt

When I decided to lose weight, and later, when I was looking to gain muscle mass, the first thing I did was to read as much as possible about the best ways to do so. Even after choosing a diet and establish a plan, I kept on reading, researching and adapting when I felt it was necessary to improve the chances of achieving my goal. I recommend you to do the same.

Always look for more than one source. Don't believe anything you have not read at least in two different places and that doesn't seem to make sense. Learn about your body, its functions and the factors that make it work. Read about food, and why it produces the reactions it produces. Don't be afraid to try new things, but do not feel the urge to try the first thing you find. Find out what can work for you and discard what doesn't. Remember, we're talking about your body and your health. If you do not care about yourself, who will?

9. Every day, do a little better

As you've already seen, this is an advice I'm giving you in every section of the book. Remember what you did yesterday (or if you write it down if it's easier) and do a little better today. Small increases every day, I ask no more. You'll see how they will make a big difference.

To end this chapter, I want to leave you with this fragment of a very interesting article about weight loss. It's called "One Weight-Loss Approach fits all? No, Not Even Close ", it was written by Gina Kolata and was published in the New York

Times on 12 December 2016. It describes weight-loss stories of several people and the various methods they used. Every one of them did it differently but the important thing was that they shared the same mentality. And that's what I want to convey to you in this book.

"Dr. Frank Sacks, a professor of nutrition at Harvard, likes to challenge his audience when he gives lectures on obesity.
"If you want to make a great discovery," he tells them, figure out this: Why do some people lose 50 pounds on a diet while others on the same diet gain a few pounds?
Then he shows them data from a study he did that found exactly that effect.
Dr. Sacks's challenge is a question at the center of obesity research today. Two people can have the same amount of excess weight, they can be the same age, the same socioeconomic class, the same race, the same gender. And yet a treatment that works for one will do nothing for the other.

The problem, researchers say, is that obesity and its precursor — being overweight — are not one disease but instead, like cancer, they are many. "You can look at two people with the same amount of excess body weight and they put on the weight for very different reasons," said Dr. Arya Sharma, medical director of the obesity program at the University of Alberta."

Time to workout

If we really want lose weight, dieting will not be enough. You need physical activity, and I know that many people don't like it, but it doesn't have to be torture. In fact, this section of the book, as in almost all others, we will talk about a gradual increase, which will make our life much easier.

Before you continue, I want to warn you about something. I have talked about exercise as a complement to your diet, and that's the way it should be seen. Unfortunately, several studies have shown working out on it's own doesn't make you lose weight.

To give some evidence to my claim I will now quote an article called "Why you shouldn't exercise to lose weight, explained with 60+ studies", that appeared on the website Vox in April 28, 2016.

The benefits of exercise are real. And stories about people who have lost a tremendous amount of weight by hitting the treadmill abound. But the bulk of the evidence tells a less impressive story.

Consider this review of exercise intervention studies, published in 2001: It found that after 20 weeks, weight loss was less than expected, and that "the amount of exercise energy expenditure had no correlation with weight loss in these longer studies."

To explore the effects of more exercise on weight, researchers have followed everybody from people training for marathons to sedentary young twins, and post-menopausal overweight and obese women who ramp up their physical activity through running, cycling, or personal training sessions. Most people in these studies typically only lost a few pounds at best, even under highly controlled scenarios where their diets were kept constant.

One very underappreciated fact about exercise is that, even when you workout, those extra calories burned only account for a tiny part of your total energy expenditure.

"In reality," said Alexxai Kravitz, a neuroscientist and obesity researcher at the National Institutes of Health, "it's only around 10 to 30 percent [of total energy expenditure] depending on the person (and excluding professional athletes that workout as a job)."

So, taking this into account, what I'd like to say is that you should definitely exercise, because it's good for your health and it serves as a fantastic complement to a dietary regime, but by no means it should be used as a substitute. If you want to lose weight, food comes first and exercise next.

It's hard to admit it but the natural state of modern man is laziness. It's no coincidence that most of the inventions of the last two centuries have been designed to make our life easier. Now we can do almost everything, even work, without leaving the 10-yard area around our couch, and if we really need to move, we just have to walk 20 steps, jump on the car and let the engine take us anywhere.

If we add that, when we are overweight, it's very common that we get depressed just by seeing ourselves in the mirror. And, like it happened to Kereem, feeling worse makes us want to do less things, stay on the couch, lay in bed until as late as possible and let life pass us by. Thus, we maintain a vicious circle. As we are overweight, we don't want to move, so we don't. As a consequence, we don't burn anything we eat, causing us to be even more overweight and want to move even less, and so on to infinity.

Therefore, the first recommendation on this book in that sense is precisely that: we must move. At the moment, I'm not talking about working out, not even a fast walk circuit, but simply to move. The key phrase here is "anything we can do ourselves, without a machine, must be done".

What do I mean? Well, it works this way. Do I need to go buy something? I'll walk, not take the car. Do I have to turn on the TV? I won't use the remote control. Do I need something from the kitchen? I won't ask my partner, parents or children, I'll rise up from my seat and take the 30 steps that separate me from my room! It sounds absurd, but these small efforts make a huge difference, and the truth is that they cost us nothing; it's just a question of simply shaking off the laziness for two minutes and activating ourselves a bit.

Now, once we have discussed the most basic part, let's go with some specific recommendations for those wishing to exercise beyond the normal movement of a busy day.

1. Choose something you like

This is essential, but sometimes we don't actually realize it. Many people go to a gym because it seems the easiest way to exercise, but they stop after a few days or weeks because that kind of workout doesn't motivate them.

In fact, the easiest way to exercise is to have fun. I really love tennis and soccer, so when I want to workout, the first thing I do is to take a racket or ball. Think of what you like and that's what you have to start doing. If you find nothing, remember what you liked as a child. Were you a good dancer? Well then start with salsa lessons! Did you like baseball? Go out with a ball and a glove or find a team where you can play. It's very important that you enjoy your workout, because then you're going to be motivated to do it again and again.

2. Make it a priority and do it regularly

We all have jobs, work, family and hobbies. For that reason (and because we are too lazy to do it), we often put exercise in the bottom of the list of our priorities. In consequence, we stop with the slightest excuse.

In this case, it must be different. Remember all that is at stake: your health, your emotional wellbeing and your self-esteem. Exercise has to be a vital part of your new life. Therefore, you have to make it a top priority.

What you must do is simply choose a time that you can devote only to workout. As I work from home writing, for me, the ideal time to exercise is in the mornings. I take tennis lessons twice a week (Tuesday and Thursday) for two hours, I go to the gym on Monday, Wednesday and Friday and I take a break on the weekend. I cancel only if I have urgent commitments and try to compensate by exercising another day or another hour, but almost never happens. In my mind it's clear to me that those are my exercise hours and I try never to sacrifice them. I recommend you do the same.

3. Try new things

I must make a confession. I hated the gym. I didn't understand how people could go lift weights again and again. It didn't seem to be fun at all. That feeling ended when I started to go and saw the results.

I am a very competitive person by nature, so I like sports like soccer or tennis, where there is a challenge and an incentive to win. In the gym, I found the same by trying to lift more weight each session. Albeit very gradually, that increase motivated me to go the next day, and still does.

So I invite you to try. Not only to go to the gym but also to practice a sport you've never practiced or even go to dance lessons or yoga. You never know what you may be attracted to until you really try. Just be careful, don't make a disproportionate effort the first time, go with the intention of discovering a new thing and having fun, there will be time to really take it seriously.

4. If you go to the gym, ask an instructor to make a routine for you

Going to the gym for the first (or second or third) time can be a very unsettling experience. There you are, completely out of shape, seeing how these giant guys lift dozens of pounds or girls with amazing bodies sprint at a speed you would never dream of.

It's very likely that you wonder, "what the hell am I doing here?" And start doing something, anything, to take away that impression. Then, when the giant finally leaves the machine, or the supermodel leaves the treadmill, you shyly approach and try to imitate what you saw them doing in the best possible way, cursing under your breath.

The same happened to me, many times, until I realized that one day they also arrived to a gym for the first time, just as intimidated as I was, and with the same insecurities. The only reason that they looked so strong and full of energy now was because they had been doing it for a longer time. And then I saw the reality in all its glory: it was not a superpower, simply a matter of practice!

So I swallowed my pride and did the right thing. When the gym instructor asked me if I needed help I said yes. And that muscular guy, who seemed completely unapproachable, turned out to be super friendly. He asked many questions about my lifestyle, diet and the goals I wanted to achieve in the gym. And then he designed a specific routine for my needs. When I thanked him, he told me it was not needed, since he was only doing his job.

And it still happened to me many times. I was on a machine, trying my best, and one of those giants approached me. I looked at him with fearful eyes but he, with all kindness, told me. "Doing the exercise this way, is going to get you hurt, let me show you the correct technique." And slowly I understood that lifting the weight was only half of the work, the other was doing it correctly.

During the following months, I decided to get rid of my shyness and ask as many questions as possible. I began to understand my body and I realized that some of the exercises that were on my routine didn't make me feel comfortable or hurt me, so I decided to replace them with similar ones, but who worked better for me.

As I am a very curious person, and I like to understand how things work, when I had free time, I read on the Internet about different types of workouts and muscle functions of the body, and gradually came to understand what was best for me.

I also realized that to have those unreal bodies, those people had to spend many hours in the gym, so to envy them wasn't worth it. My priority was just to stay in good shape and have a body with which I felt happy, and finally achieved my purpose. In fact, from time to time it happens to me to see someone new in the gym watching me with the same face of shyness and distrust when I'm doing an exercise. And of course, I always approach them with my best smile to try to help them feel more comfortable there. Ultimately, not too long ago I was exactly in the same position!

5. If you're going to workout, do your best!

I do not know who it was, but someone once said "no pain no gain", and the phrase was marked forever among those who workout. I agree with it, but obviously figuratively! In my opinion, if you're going to do sport you have to put maximum effort. Otherwise, what's the use?

In the gym, there's nothing that bothers me more than to see those people who go just to brag that they spent an hour doing sport, but sit on a stationary bike and pedal slowly while sending Whatsapp messages and take selfies.

That's not only a waste of time, but they are deceiving themselves, and if you paid attention, that's the worst possible thing in my book. If you decide to do a sport, do your best! Not only for your health but also because exercise releases endorphins, which will make you feel better, much more than if you sit on a bike to check the Facebook updates to a cousin that you haven't seen since 20 years ago.

7. Each day, make it a little better

When I got my first routine in the gym, the first thing I did was record how much I lifted in each of the exercises, so it would be easy to remember me the next time I had to do a particular exercise. Besides, that way I could slowly measure my improvement, and that helped my motivation over time.

Now there are really useful apps that make your life easier, whether in the gym, running or even to count the steps you take each day. I will not recommend any in particular because they are all very similar, all you have to do is go to your AppStore and find the one that appeals more to you.

Measuring your progress is very important and, as I told you earlier in the book, the key to lose weight and live a healthier life is to remember what you did yesterday and do a little better today. Small increases every day, I ask no more. You'll see how they will make a big difference.

The right mindset to lose weight

This is the last section of the book, and certainly the most important. Unlike others who have written on the subject, the most important thing for me to lose weight are not the techniques you follow but the mentality that you have during the process. If your mind is on the right track I guarantee you will loss weight.

1. Stop lying to yourself

Being fat is not OK! It's not! Period! That last piece of pizza will indeed make a difference. Stopping in the middle of your workout routine is not the same than finishing it. Society is not to blame. There is always time to exercise. You don't have an injury. Obese people have a lower life expectancy. It doesn't matter if you have work/school/children. You don't need to spend a fortune in order to workout. Tell yourself this every day and leave the excuses! You know they are not true and that all you're doing is lying to yourself and letting down your loved ones. Think what's at stake, your health and mental wellbeing. Is there anything more important than that?

2. Find your "enough is enough" moment

I will begin this section by quoting a post of a Reddit user, Rafiki, which perfectly explains the concept of "enough is enough"

"Five years ago I weighed 340 lbs. I had high blood pressure, high cholesterol, chest pains, swollen ankles, sleep apnea... pretty much all the health issues associated with being obese. On top of it all I suffered from major depressive episodes and had no friends so I isolated myself in my bedroom and just hoped I'd have a heart attack one day and die.

One afternoon my mom called from the living room asking if I could help her with the TV because she wanted to record her favorite show while dad was watching his news so after a few minutes of grumbling I came out and grabbed the remote and set the DVR to record her show and gave it back to her and before returning to my room she turned around and said:

"Thanks, son, I don't know what we'll do if you're not around to help us with these things."

Now I've been obese most of my life and I've been on the receiving end of countless lectures, advice, and ridicule but none of them affected me the way this statement did. It planted a seed in my mind that sprouted and turned into something I thought was never possible. I was now concerned about my well being, not because I wanted to look better, but because I didn't want my mother to have to bury her own son".

To Rafiki, the "enough is enough" moment was to realize how important he was for their parents; for me, it was seeing a video of me and not recognizing the guy who was on the screen, to Kereem it was moving to Europe and discover that most men were more attractive than him. We've all had our "enough is enough" moments that have changed our lives.

Obviously, it's difficult to artificially generate one of these moments, because we all have our own process. Every person I have mentioned in this section took years to reach the point of really wanting to change, and it's likely that it won't happen immediately to you, but what I want to ask you now is to be open to the possibility.

How to do it? Think about the things you want, what you've always dreamed of, the people you love and what would happen if you wouldn't be with them. The moments you have missed and that will never come back. The moments you will have in the future and let escape if you don't something about it. Get ready for the time when your mind says, "enough is enough", and once that happens, do not look back. Your life depends on it.

3. Understands that the road doesn't always go in a straight line

As I said in the previous section, all the people I know who have lost weight had to follow a long process, which was never as easy as it seemed. Sometimes we lose pounds and then recover them. Sometimes our discipline fails us. Sometimes something happens in our life that makes us falter.

The road never goes in a straight line, and it's very normal that your weight will fluctuate up and down on the way to having the body you want to have. What's important is that you understand it, not be too hard on yourself and stay on the road, even if there are some detours. If we make a chart of how your weight loss should be, it should look more or less like this.

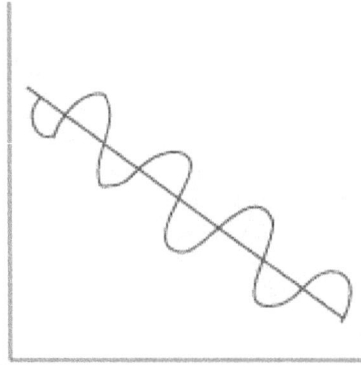

As you see, the idea is that there is always a downhill tendency, although there are ups and downs along the way.

4. Measure, understand and adapt

We all know that the best way to understand any topic is getting as much information as possible; however, very rarely we apply it to ourselves!

In any weight loss process, information is key. There are three main elements that have to be measured at least every week: the first, and most important, it is your body mass index (BMI). I say it is the most important because, as you will read in the next point, that's the one that will tell you whether you're on track, and if you can relax or if you have to pick up the pace. The other two are your weight and measurements of your body. I don't have to explain much why you have to weigh yourself, but the measurements are very important because, especially if you go to the gym, it's the only way to realize that even if your weight is stable, you are making significant progress. Ultimately a pound is a pound either fat or muscle, but definitely not look the same!

5. The ideal indicator to know if you're on track

On March 18, 2016, the prestigious medical magazine The Lancet published a study conducted by Dr. Richard Peto of Oxford University on the impact of obesity on life expectancy of people. The study, which tracked 894.576 people, mostly in the US and Western Europe, from 1979 to date, compared how the Body Mass Index (BMI) is correlated with mortality.

The results were not only very revealing, but they gave us the perfect indicator of whether we have a normal weight or need to do something about it. Let's read an excerpt.

"A BMI of 18.5 to 24.9 is normal (that translates to weighing between 114 and 149 pounds if you're 5 feet 5 inches tall); overweight is 25 to 29.9 (150 to 179 pounds if you're 5 feet 5 inches tall); and obese is 30 or more (180 pounds-plus on a 5-

foot-5-inch frame.) You can figure out your BMI at the National Institutes of Health Web site.

Men and women in the new analysis who had BMIs between 22.5 and 25 were the least likely to die during the follow-up period, which averaged eight years. But every additional 5 BMI points boosted mortality risk by 30 percent. The increase was strongest for deaths due to cardiovascular disease, diabetes, kidney, and liver disease; cancer deaths also went up with increasing BMI, but not as much as other diseases. The researchers calculate that having a BMI of 30 to 35 takes to two to four years off the average lifespan compared with having a BMI of 22.5 to 25. Having a BMI between 40 and 45 (for example, being 5 feet 5' and weighing 240 to 270 pounds), they say, reduces one's lifespan by eight to 10 years. This reduction in lifespan is on par with being a heavy smoker."

There is the information, and now the question: do you want to die young, probably in a horrible way and to leave your loved ones? If the answer is no (and I hope it is! Otherwise, it's time to seek professional help right now), it is time to take action.

What should you do? Measure your BMI using these formulas:

Measurement Units	Formula and Calculation
Kilograms and meters (or centimeters)	Formula: weight (kg) / [height (m)]^2
	With the metric system, the formula for BMI is weight in kilograms divided by height in meters squared. Because height is commonly measured in centimeters, divide height in centimeters by 100 to obtain height in meters.
	Example: Weight = 68 kg, Height = 165 cm (1.65 m)
	Calculation: 68 ÷ (1.65)^2 = 24.98
Pounds and inches	Formula: weight (lb) / [height (in)]^2 x 703
	Calculate BMI by dividing weight in pounds (lbs) by height in inches (in) squared and multiplying by a conversion factor of 703.
	Example: Weight = 150 lbs, Height = 5'5" (65")
	Calculation: [150 ÷ (65)^2] x 703 = 24.96

Source: Centers for Disease Control and Prevention

Now you have your number. If you are between 18.5 and 24.9, congratulations! You're a normal person. Of course, you may still want to lose (or gain) a little weight and follow the advice in this book, but you shouldn't be too worried. If you have more than that number, it's time to start a diet and increase your exercise level.

Make this calculation every month. If you see that your BMI is already in normal parameters, you rest easy, if not, you should stick with the diet. Easy peasy! Isn't it?

Just a clarification. BMI doesn't measure the difference between fat and muscle, so if you're following an exercise protocol to gain mass, it won't give you an accurate result. In such a case, the ideal thing is to buy one of those scales that tell you what percentage of body fat you have. The normal range is between 14 and 17 as a man, and between 21 and 24 as a woman.

6. Losing weight is a marathon, not a 100-yard race

Any diet that proposes miraculous results in a few days is either lying or dangerous to your health (or both). The goal should be to lose weight and feel good, even if it represents a longer-term effort. I'll tell you now, your path will be complicated, with ups and downs, moments of great joy and others of great frustration. Do not lose patience! As I showed in the graph in the last chapter, the important thing is to stay on the right path.

7. Yes, you're beautiful, no matter what they say, but you can always be a better version of yourself.

This is the last paragraph of the book, and perhaps the most important. We are all beautiful, but we all also have the potential to be better. You do not have to look up to any model or a Hollywood actor. Your challenge is to surpass yourself, and become your best version. Behind that person you see in the mirror today there is a much better one ready to emerge at the moment that you decide. Do it today, because tomorrow may be too late.